God Must Think I'm A Bad Ass

A Short Novel By:
Essence Unique

Foreward:

To my person, the first person to show me unconditional love, the best person that is always there. And my everything, I could never say it enough but Thank you. I love you . Know I wouldn't have gotten this far without you. Here's to you mommy….

Names of doctor's and some hospitals have been changed.

Chapter One

"Endurance is not just the ability to bear a hard thing, but to turn it into a glory"- William Barclay

They say God gives his toughest battles to his strongest soldiers. Well God must think I'm a Bad Ass. Because for the past few years I have been living through the toughest battle of my life. Between me and you I don't know if I'm winning this battle like a Bad Ass, but at least i'm winning. Let's start from the beginning. On October 29th,2014 one day after my 20th birthday I went to my yearly optometrist visit just to get my eyes checked. I had cancelled said appointment twice already due to work but I needed to go.Little did I know that would be one of the worst days of my life. At first the appointment started off as any other. I picked out some new glasses, took the vision test and the doctor dilated my pupils. As I am waiting, the doctor came in and ask me if I want to try this new test for free on this new machine he had. This machine takes pictures of the back of the eye and gives information doctors can't see from just looking at your eye. I don't know what made me agree, but I did.

I took the test and Dr.Kramer sits me back in the room while he goes and get the pictures. Twenty minutes goes by with no doctor…. Forty minutes goes by and still no doctor. Now I'm getting antsy, I have to be in class in an hour. After an hour of waiting Dr.Kramer comes in and I can instantly tell by the look on his face that something is wrong. He says "Ms.Cheatom, I seen some abnormalities in your pictures" "well what is it Dr.Kramer don't keep me waiting" I say. He responds while putting pictures up on the screen " Looks like you have a condition called Pseudotumor Cerebri, that just means there is swelling in your optic nerves.Im going to send you to a specialist that I know can help you." So many things are running through my mind. One my vision has been changing so much and so fast now I know why. Two did my epilepsy cause this? Should I have known that something was wrong? Why did I cancel my appointments before? I am more scared then I have ever been in my life. Tears are running marathons down my face. I try my hardest to collect myself so I can get to my car and go home..

I call my mom and tearfully try to explain what Dr.Kramer just told me, as confused as I was she lets me know everything is going to be okay and that she will call the doctor and get more information. Driving home in tears was hard enough for me, so I'm going to skip class today and get myself together. Who would've known that missing class that day would be the first time of many for me. Shane my boyfriend meets me at my house because as expected I am a complete mess. My mom calls back and tells me the doctor said its not as awful as it may have seemed and to not worry until we meet with the doctor. We would soon learn that it was awful and we had a lot to worry about and most importantly it would not be okay, not for awhile.

I will never know what made this stupid disease kick into gear but a couple days after diagnosis I started having terrible headaches and my vision continually got worse. Everyday my mom was calling to see if the specialist could fit us in. While waiting for that appointment seeing in class was getting harder, driving to and from work was difficult and those headaches, boy were they debilitating.But I could not just stop everything.I had a life, I had dreams and goals I could not let this stop me not yet.

On the 4th of November I was working the election. Against the advice of my mom, Shane and my body I went and worked the election anyway. 14 of the longest hours of my life. Looking back I don't know how I finished the day, but I did. I would pay for it the next day though. November 5th sitting in my english class at Ohio Dominican I had a seizure. Me having seizures was not uncommon as I had been diagnosed with epilepsy earlier in the year. I have been having seizures since 2009 and had experienced some bad ones. But this seizure was worse, Im sure it was my bodies reaction from being in so much pain and simply being exhausted. A trip to the hospital and some rest is all I needed. A couple hours of rest and some fluids and home I go.

Two weeks later we finally got an appointment with a specialist I had never heard of, a Neuro-Opthamologist. His name is Dr.Elias and he explains that Pseudotumor Cerebri is a condition where excess Spinal Fluid builds up on and around your brain. When this happens it causes your optic nerves to swell affecting your vision. Its symptoms include headaches, body pain, swooshing in the ear, balance and gait issues ,nausea and vomiting. Pseudotumor Cerebri is more recently called Intracranial Hypertension because the increased fluid on your brain, increases the pressure in your brain. The kind I have was Idiopathic because we will never know why, how or even when I had contracted it. Great just like me to get another rare condition. Did I forget to mention that we learned that day that Pseudotumor is also not curable only manageable.Hearing that I have to deal with this for the rest of my life was crushing. Dr.Elias thinks that this "wonderful" medicine called Diamox would help me but first he wanted me to have a Spinal tap.A spinal tap also called a Lumbar Puncture is a procedure a radiologist performs where they take spinal fluid from your spine in your lower back with a very large and long needle.At this point during my battle I am more than afraid I am Petrified.

Just four days later me, my mom and shane are on our way to the hospital for my very first spinal tap. Never would have thought that now four years later I would have experienced more spinal taps than I could count. The radiologist said it wouldn't be painful but I was not looking forward to having that long needle stuck in my spine.And he lied because it did hurt, It hurt so freaking much! Oh my goodness I had never felt anything like that. A couple hours later Im home and two days later we are back in Dr.Elias's office. He tells us that normal spinal fluid pressure is between 8 and 15 but that it fluctuates, if it goes above 20 thats when you are diagnosed with Pseudotumor Cerebri. My Pressure was 48, that was over twice the amount that it should've been. Now I feel like why me God? What am I going to do now? Dr.Elias continues to tell me how bad my vision is now and says that I need yet another specialist a Surgical Neuro Opthamologist to help me

manage since my pressure was so high. He prescribes the diamox and says that should lower my pressure and help while we wait for an appointment to the next doctor. I can't help but think damn here we go again, just like when I started having seizures. I went to doctor after doctor. No one wanted to help me, no one could help me, no one believed me. It was always more hurry up and wait, more of being passed on and forgotten about, another medicine thats not going to work, more pain and less vision,more of our time wasted.I felt exhausted already.

While waiting on the appointment I started the diamox which as falsely advertised was the devil. After a day of taking it, my tongue was numb, I couldn't taste carbonation and my lips, toes, and fingers were tingling like pins and needles. But I took it as prescribed because I would do anything to get rid of this headache. Nothing helped not motrin, not advil, not aleve, not sleep, not this Diamox NOTHING took this pounding headache away. I could hear my heartbeat in my ear the swooshing overtone was annoying and it felt as if my brain was going to explode. I couldn't see enough to drive anymore and my grades in school were worsening.I had already taken a leave of absence from work until I was better.All of my energy was in going to class and trying not to succumb to the pain.

The new specialist, Dr.Benett was great, after seeing my test results she got me in quickly and was very nice. Her office was in the same building as Dr.Elias's and when I left I felt like she would help me as much as she could. She told me the diamox wasn't working and since it was making sick I should stop taking it. She did extensive test and told us just how bad my vision was becoming, she told me that the pressure in my eye was still extremely high despite the diamox and that in a few days Id probably be blind. She let me know that it was probably a good time to leave school for awhile and that I would need to have a shunt placed to drain the fluid. A shunt is just a plastic tube that can be placed in your spine and drains in your

stomach and that is called an LP Shunt or Lumbar Peritoneal Shunt. There is also a VP Shunt or Ventriculoperitoneal Shunt that is placed in your brain and drains in your stomach.Dr.Benett suggested I needed a VP Shunt and also that if my vision got worse in the next couple of days that I should go to the E.R. and have an emergency Spinal tap. She sent my file to neurosurgeons at different hospitals in the city to see who could fit me in the soonest. One said they had met their Shunt quota for the year and couldn't help me. The other said that he didn't have anytime until february to place my shunt, it was the 2nd of december, and I'll be completely blind before then. We leave Dr.Benett office with her promising to find the right surgeon to help me as soon as possible.As I said I knew she would help in every way she could and she did.

In denial I still tried to go to school everyday as if nothing was wrong. I was sitting in the front of the class not seeing anything my professor was writing on the board. Missing important things and only hearing the whooshing in my ears. I kept up the facade for a few more days until I got a test back that I got a 3 out of 18 on. I knew the material I thought.I had studied for this test. But it is hard to study material if you wrote the wrong things down because you couldn't see or hear the material. I had never been a failing student so that realization stung, like hell. In that moment, gazing at that test I decided it was time to take leave of absence from school. I cried filling out the paperwork.

God works in mysterious ways though because while my mom was taking me out shopping and to dinner to try and cheer me up that evening, a Nurse Practitioner working for a NeuroSurgeon at The Ohio State University Wexner Medical Center called us.She tells us that they seen my file and want me to come to the E.R. to be admitted. Her boss a neuroSurgeon didn't think it was safe for me to be anywhere other than the hospital with pressure that high. If your pressure gets to high you can have a brain hemorrhage, a

stroke and even die. Her doctor was out of town tonight but he would place my shunt as soon as he returned. We left shopping and made our way home to pack. A couple hours later we were in the E.R. All these different doctors came in to see me. I had to take another vision test and do blood work. I had MRI'S, XRAY,CT SCANS and an MRV done. MRI is Magnetic Resonance Imaging. For Pseudotumor they use this imaging to see if Doctors can find any excess fluid in your skull. X RAYS are electromagnetic images as well that show structural damages to your skull and later in my case my shunt systems.The CT Scan or computed tomography scan takes a lot of pictures like from x rays and creates cross sectional images so that doctors can see inside of areas without cutting. MRV is a test just like an MRI but it uses dye so light up the veins in your body so doctors know just where they are and if they are under or over sized,After all of those test and before finally admitting me they wanted to do a bedside Spinal Tap to see what my pressure was currently. Whoa I thought the first one hurt this one was horrendous. It took them 6 sticks and 2 doctors to draw fluid from my spine. My boyfriend and Uncle in the hall were ready to beat up the doctor because they could hear me screaming down the hall. After finally drawing fluid my pressure was still 48 and I was legally blind. The neurosurgery team decided I couldn't wait for that doctor to come back in town I needed to have a shunt placed soon. I was admitted to the hospital December 5th and the next day at 4pm I had my very first Surgery.

Chapter Two

"Sometimes the things we can't change end up changing us"-Unknown

Doctors had told us that once I got a shunt everything would be fine. My headaches would go away, my vision gets better and I wouldn't have to worry about the shunt anymore. Well we soon learned that, that was a lie. On December 6th they placed a programmable shunt in my spine called an LP shunt. It pumps the excess fluid on my brain and diverts it down my spine where it empties into my stomach. I thought the pain from that surgery was the worst thing I would ever feel in my life but I soon learned that too was not going to be the case.

After four days in the hospital I was able to go home. My family and I were relieved beyond measure. The pain was so bad I couldn't even turn to wipe my own butt.That was the most humbled and embarrassed I had been but I knew I had to get through this pain, heal up and get back to school, work and my life.Everyday I put all my energy into getting better. Slowly but surely my vision was coming back and I felt a little bit better everyday. Week four of my healing comes along and I feel well enough to go on a date with my man. He took me out to lunch and to the movies. I was so excited because for the first time since diagnosis I had hope. Hope that I would be normal again and that Id live a full life again without headaches,without pain.But On week eight while sitting in church I noticed this pulling pain in my neck, as church goes on a headache starts and it gets worse by the minute. This new headache was much different than the headache I had before surgery. It wasn't only different but much worse. Later that night it was still bothering me. Everytime I set up even to just go pee or change positions in bed my brain felt like it was coming out of the back of my skull. Ugh it was terrible. I thought to myself "damn I can't even enjoy church anymore without this condition interrupting." Just when I started to have hope that things would get better they start getting worse. I get a little bit of my life back and just as quickly as it came its snatched away from me. Monday we go to the doctor, they try to delicately explain that these things can happen and my shunt probably just needs to be adjusted. I smile and nod in agreeance but deep down I know we are nowhere near the end of this hellish battle.They adjusted my shunt and we went home. No change with the headache after a couple days so back to the doctor we go. The shunt is adjusted again. As you can probably guess by now there was no change after the adjustment. We had to go to the doctor four more times for adjustments and still No change.

Currently I am miserable, frustrated and hurting. My vision is stable but everything else is in shambles. Despite the four adjustments to my shunt I am still having what doctor's call low pressure headaches. My shunt is working to well and draining to much fluid, the pulling of the fluid down through my spine is what's causing the headaches. Let's be honest it's head pain because there is no headache that feels this bad. Anyway the low pressure headache goes away when I lay down and feels better when I drink caffeine but how much caffeine can you drink? You can't lay down all day everyday but that's what the doctor wants me to do until they figure out how to fix me. Two weeks go by and I can not take it anymore I walk into the doctor appointment with my mom and let him have a piece of my mind. I demanded a new doctor, someone with more experience. Someone that can help me. Surprisingly the doctor and his nurse agreed that we needed to bring someone else in who was a better fit for me. They set me up with an appointment to see one of the best Neurosurgeons in Columbus Dr.John McConnel. Dr.McConnel handles about 90% of the Pseudotumor Cerebri cases in Ohio. Although I knew seeing a new doctor meant getting comfortable with someone else, a lot more test and maybe even another surgery I was excited to get a doctor who listens to me.

We were able to see the new doctor a couple weeks later and he was great. Dr.McConnel was soft spoken but firm and had a bedside manner like I had never experienced. He explained that they would do more test as I expected, an MRI, CT Scan and Spinal tap. In the meantime he said I should keep drinking the caffeine when I need to be upright. So I did what he said anytime I had a doctor's appointment, physical therapy session or out with family I drank caffeine. By the time of my Spinal tap I was drinking almost a 2 liter of Mountain Dew a day. The spinal tap and all the other test confirmed what we already knew that I was having low pressure headaches. What the test can not confirm is why the settings of my shunt wont stop the overdraining. I mean that's what the different shunt settings are supposed to do. Dr.McConnel explains to us that I might need another shunt in my brain this time though to lessen the pull of my brain down my spine. The shunts would work together to give me some relief and hopefully work together to give me normal spinal fluid pressure, finally. After that appointment with him I felt like I had just met the man who would save my life. Dr.McConnel had to go out of town to teach for awhile but as soon as he got back he would perform my surgery. At this point I feel informed, Im not scared just ready to fight, hopeful that this solution would be the key for me to get better. I guess that's the type of confidence a good doctor can instill in his patients.The placement of the new shunt would mean shaving my head so before this condition could take my hair like it did everything else, I tried to take power back into my own hands by cutting my hair. I hated the haircut but at least I had done it, not the doctor, I was not going to let this condition take one more thing from me.I drank almost a 2 liter of caffeine from the day of the appointment until March 23rd,2015 when I had my second surgery but my first brain surgery.

This is going to sound crazy but the brain surgery was easier than the first surgery. I couldn't believe how quick my recovery was. I was in the hospital for 3 days but I started feeling better as soon as I got home. It felt so good to not have head pain again. I was anxious that like last time the better feelings would not last long but even so I couldn't maintain my excitement. I went back to church, I was doing housework again and going out looking cute with my man. I just knew I was better. I wasn't even worried about the new ugly hairstyle I had.I just knew I was better.

But better only lasted about 8 weeks. Not only had my LP Shunt broken but my Vp Shunt was clogged. My vision was declining rapidly and I was always in pain.We had been back and forth to the doctor every 2 or 3 days having my shunts adjusted. Nothing and I mean nothing was working. It happened out of nowhere, I was watching movies with my niece one saturday when my I heard the dreaded ringing and swooshing in my ear. I knew that meant my spinal fluid pressure was high. My face and body had started swelling as well. Everything was going to hell and quickly. On a busy day of doctor appointments I found out I needed to have a very difficult surgery where they would fix both of my shunts at the same time. I would have to wait about a month because again my doctor has to go out of town. On the same dreaded day my eye doctor Dr.Benett informs me that I will be blind in about a month and suggest that I have an eye surgery to save my vision while we're waiting for my other surgery.That surgery is called a Double Nerve Sheath Decompression. She would have to take my eyeballs out of my brain and cut slits throughout my optic nerves so that the excess spinal fluid can drain through those slits instead of building up and swelling my optic nerves. What a Shit day right? Not only do I find out that I have to have another brain and spinal surgery in a couple months, I have to have an eye surgery before that because i'm going blind. I am so emotional right now. All I can do is cry. Im petrified and physically and emotionally exhausted.

Chapter Three

"Although the world is full of suffering,it is also full of the overcoming of it"-Helen Keller

It's the morning of June 17th and I'm hungry from not being able to eat since before midnight. Also i'm nervous but relieved that with my eye surgery I don't have to stay in the hospital. We get to the surgery center and its showtime.Before my surgeries to calm me down I look at all the pictures in my phone and relive beautiful moments. The double Nerve Sheath Decompression I had was fairly quick, but for my eyes to heal Id actually be blind for a couple of days. When I woke up all I see is darkness, although I expected the darkness I didn't expect how final it feels. I hear my moms and Shane's voice and instantly it calms me. I couldn't wait to get home and for these 2 days of darkness to be over.After sleeping off the sedation and my family visiting me at home, I don't remember much else of the next few days. Only thing I really remember is the darkness and taking the bandages off of my eyes.Seeing the faces of my loved ones was reassuring, I would never not want to be able to see their beautiful faces again. A week later we went back to the eye doctor and she made sure that everything was okay. My vision seemed to be better, now I just have to wait for my next surgery. I have 19 days left, only 19 days until relief again, I can make it.

19 days later I did get relief. It came after having the hardest surgery to date for me. After they fixed my Lp Shunt, They turned me over and unclogged my VP Shunt. I was in the hospital for 5 days and I was in so much pain. None of the medicine seemed to help enough and I don't remember anything from my time in the hospital other than the pain. It seemed like nothing but pain until I woke up at home. I was at managing at home and after about 2 weeks I feeling better than I had felt since I was diagnosed. When I say better I mean I better. My vision was stable finally, my glasses were working finally and I had found some wigs to make me look cute while my hair grew back .I even felt well enough to try and go back to work!

Chapter Four

"Difficult roads often lead to Beautiful destinations"-Unknown

I was looking for work and hopeful that it would come soon. I hadn't worked in 7 months and leaving the workforce the way I did I knew it would be hard for me to explain to a potential employer. I wanted a job where I could help people and I needed a job where I could sit most of the time or not have to do physical labor. I was somewhat healthy now but I did not want to do to much too fast, so I kept looking. Eventually I found a job as a registration representative at a local hospital.. After a couple weeks of phone interviews and shadowing I got the job. A job where I could help others and could sit most of the day.A job I had a different perspective at since I was a professional patient now and spent a lot of my time in hospitals. I was so happy, I knew this was the first step in getting my life back on track. I felt needed again and I was more than happy to have some responsibility back in my life.

My mom told me before I started that even though the doctors had cleared me to work that she felt it was too soon.She thought that I should have given it more time. I've always been head strong and nothing ever stopped from getting something I wanted. And I wanted to work, but I should've listened to my mom because after only 2 months and 20 days my illness came back with a vengeance. This time was a little different. It wasn't just my ears swooshing that told me something was wrong but it was hard for me to walk. I would be walking and my right leg would just give out. I was again in so much pain. My vision was going bad as well. I was reading a patient's insurance information and it all blurred, My new friend at work was helping me out but I knew it would only get worse. So I went back to the doctor. We went through all the normal questions and test and the doctor didn't know why I was having this pain in my back and why my leg was giving out. Of course I insisted that I knew something was wrong and one of these test was going to prove it. Days and days went by with my vision worsening daily, something was really wrong and they had better figure it out quickly or I would go blind. Finally my Ct Scan test results are back and it's time to go see the doctor. I take off early from work and hobble my way across the street where I meet my mom for my appointment. Normally when we go to see Dr.McConnel and his nurse Jane meet us in a patient room down the hall from their office, this time he ask for us to come to his office to talk. My heart instantly drops because

I know nothing good is going to come from this appointment. I prepare for the worse but pray for the best. Nothing could prepare me though for what he was about to tell us. He says my Lp Shunt in my spine has broken in 3 places and those pieces are floating around my spinal canal. I have to have an emergency Laminectomy where he will surgically remove the back of one or more of my vertebrae to get to my spinal canal and try to remove the pieces and relieve pressure from my nerves. Then they'd place another shunt. Wow, how does this keep happening to me? Did I break my shunt? It has to be something that I am doing that this keeps happening, right? Why me Lord, another surgery only 3 months after my last one? I'm thinking my body cant take much more than this. Then my mind goes to work, what am I going to do about this job? It's 3pm on a friday and I'm having surgery on monday. In 2 days. Stuff like this only happens to me.

Anyway no matter what I am thinking or how I feel I have to do what needs to be done. I call and leave messages for my bosses explaining my situation. I do all that I can to prepare for this surgery on such short notice. Monday comes rather quickly but I'm ready because this surgery means I'll be able to walk again. Monday morning comes and into surgery I go. After a long 4 hour surgery I am in a room and in excruciating pain. Every inch of my body hurts. I have never felt anything like this in my life. My back muscles feel like they have been pulled apart. No amount of sedation could help this and the pain medicine and muscle relaxers aren't helping.On top of all of that this anti-nausea medicine is making me projectile vomit. I think I will be able to go home in a couple days until the physical therapist comes in the room. She wants me to get up and try to walk, as she is helping me out of bed I realize I cant use my right leg.. The doctors had told Shane and my mom that one of the pieces of my shunt was wrapped around the nerves that control my right leg. If the feeling and motion didn't come back in a few days I might have to go to a rehab facility. There was no way I wanted that so I worked harder than I ever had so that I could go home. After 5 days my right leg still wasn't working properly but they let me go home, as long as I did at home physical therapy. Reluctantly I agreed and thankfully I went home. Two days later the home nurse and physical therapist started coming to our house. I know they were there to help but I just wanted to rest, to be alone, to try and get better,to go back to work.

Chapter Five

"If opening your eyes,or getting out of bed, or holding a spoon, or combing your hair is the daunting Mount everest you can climb today, that is okay"-Carmen Ambrosio

Days turned into weeks and weeks turned into months of the therapist coming to my house working with me. The two therapist I had were sweet. They were patient with me and understood the pain I was in. They pushed me HARD but not harder than I could handle. I was grateful for them but also grateful when they said their time was up and there was nothing else they could do for me.Sad that I hadn't progressed enough for them to continue but grateful because I could have some peace and quiet in my house and I could get some rest. But them leaving means I still don't have full use of my right leg and now I have to start outpatient physical therapy twice a week. Dr.McConnel says that maybe Water therapy will help me get better faster and relieve the pain and tingling from my nerves. A couple days later I started aqua therapy at a local hospital here in Columbus,Ohio. My new therapist was amazing. I had never had a therapist be so compassionate but stern at the same time. Her name was Jessica and she was a Neuro Therapist. A Neurotherapist does physical and occupational therapy for people who deal specifically with Neurological conditions. She worked to not just strengthen my right leg but my spine and she also worked on my balance and everything in between. The water therapy was really helping, after months I slowly got stronger and better. I went from being confined to a wheelchair when I started Aqua Therapy to walking with a walker. After using the walker for months I still continued to get stronger and I went on to start walking with a rollator. I know it's just a walker with a seat but it made me excited, it gave me more freedom. At this point in my battle I had accepted that I probably wouldn't be going back to work soon but I was feeling better and that had to be enough.

As I am sure you can guess by now I never went back to work. I did continue getting better though. From November 2nd,2015 until about April of 2016 I was better. I was walking on a cane, I was gardening and having fun again. I didn't have headaches anymore and for the most part my vision was stable.Stable vision still means blurriness,not being able to see in the dark and blind spots but I wasn't blind.I still went to physical therapy twice a week and sometimes had to go see my neurosurgeon but I was good. Until that dreaded day when I realized I had not felt or heard my Vp Shunt in my brain drain.

On top of my shunt not draining, when I would stand up I would have low pressure headaches that were starting to get worse. It was odd though because when I would lay down I would still have high pressure headaches. I didn't know what was happening or why for that matter. I felt myself falling back into that never ending circle. As soon as my life starts getting back on track, as soon as I am a little better my illness takes it all away. Here I am once again dragging my ass back to the doctors office.

As per Usual my doctors don't know why I am having problems again. Apparently there is nothing to explain my symptoms. So we go through the normal test to see if they can find the problem and still nothing. .My break down moment comes after a spinal tap. The radiologist performing it, tells me my opening pressure is 19. Now that's normal so I should be excited but Im not. I break down in tears still laying on the table. I've never had symptoms that couldn't be explained by my test results. I felt like my body was lying to me. I felt like I was going crazy. What was I going to do now? My doctors would not do anything to fix me if they didn't think that anything was wrong. Back to being miserable is all I could think about. How long would it last this time? Flustered I pulled myself together so my mom wouldn't see me cry. I think she knew though because I could see it on her face when she walked in the recovery room. I still remember that touch she gave me. Her simply pushing my hair back behind my ear relaxed me. As much as I tried to fight it I broke down in her arms.

Chapter Six

"Courage is not having the strength to go on; it is going on when you don't have the strength."-Theodore Roosevelt

I cried and cried until it was time to go home. I felt shitty for days, I didn't understand anything that was happening. My body was telling me that something was wrong but none of the normal test could prove it. Nothing was helping me and everyday my pain seemed to get worse. I started doing research to try and figure out something, anything. I found this test called ICP Bolt Monitoring. In this test doctors will surgically place a bolt in my skull that will monitor my pressures and see what each shunt is doing so we can figure out what needs to be done for me. I decided I would bring it up to my doctor at my next appointment. And I did, Dr.McConnel tells me that not only does he still not know what is wrong with me but that he does not perform that test. He said because it has never gave him many answers and it is too expensive. Damn my shitty mood just got even worse.I don't care how much it cost I just want to feel better. I can't stop the tears from flowing.I know something is wrong with my body.

I was sad for days, I cried for days, my heart broke over and over again every time I thought about my situation. I felt hopeless and at a point of no return. I didn't know I would ever be okay but Shane, my mom even my 9 year old niece in all her wisdom knew. So I had to be okay to give them hope. I guess at the time I just didn't know that doing it for them meant i was doing it for me too. Looking in her eyes while we ate breakfast after church stopped my tears. Her dreams of me at her wedding in the future stopped my tears, it made me realize that even in these bad times, in this bad battle I am still blessed, I am a blessing to her and I needed to start fighting for myself again,fighting for my nieces and nephews and little cousins who look up to me. Giving up, feeling sad and sorry for myself wasn't an option I had to be a blessing again.For them.

My tears had stopped and I was fighting every second to feel better. but it didn't stop my fear. The fear of not knowing what was wrong.Despite my doctors not knowing what was wrong with me either I kept making appointments to go back. I was going to make them see me, make them feel my pain until they tried to fix me. Hell I would just settle for them to research a solution. While I continued calling and going to the doctor I did my own research. I researched the best hospitals for my condition, the best doctors and ways that I could go see them. I wanted to make sure that I could say that I did everything in my power to get better. After bringing the information I found to my mom and Shane we decided to go to one of the hospitals I had found Cleveland Clinic. There was a doctor there named Dr.Lucca that I wanted to see. He is a NeuroSurgeon that specializes in Pseudotumor Cerebri, one of the best in his field. I had read stories from people whose lives he saved and I knew if I could get a second opinion from him then I'd start on the right path.

But you can't just go to a new Neurosurgeon in a different city, you have to send in a bunch of information and they will then decide if they will accept your case. While gathering the information though I still needed to go to the doctor here. After switching both my shunt settings what felt like a thousand times there was still no relief. So my doctor decided to try a new pump called an Anti-Siphon Valve. This valve would be attached to my LP Shunt. It would give me more range instead of just one setting. Hopefully the valve would stop the low pressure headaches when I am standing up and the high pressure headaches when Im laying down. Not many people in the world have this valve and I would be the first one to have it attached to an LP shunt. My doctor had never placed this valve before .He was using me as a test dummy and I was terrified by that, but also I felt important. If this treatment worked for me, it might help hundreds of people who endure this battle just like me. Unfortunately though I would have to wait AGAIN for my surgery because Dr.McConnel was going out of town. Only 2 weeks this time but 2 weeks full of pain. Two weeks later on May 19th,2016 I had my sixth surgery.

The sixth surgery was by far the easiest. I only spent one night in the hospital. After a couple weeks of healing I went back to physical therapy which helped me start feeling better. I wasn't having headaches and my ears were not ringing which was a big relief. Even Though I wasn't well enough to work or even stay a home by myself yet I was okay and that was enough for me.

I enjoyed the upcoming summer. Shane taught me all about fishing and I fell in love with that. We spent time with all the little ones in our families and went on vacation. My garden I planted flourishing and I enjoyed watching what I had planted grow.Life was stable for the time being, so life was good for us. My mom was enjoying herself a little more too and my puppy was growing super fast. The thing I dreaded most happened in september. Sitting in a movie with Shane when my head starts pounding. Boom,Boom,Boom,Boom is all I can hear or feel over the movie Sully playing on the big screen. We were sitting unusually close to the screen,thinking that was the culprit of my headache I force my fears away and try to enjoy the rest of my date.. When I get home I keep avoiding my thoughts and try to rest.

Im resting until swoosh, swoosh swishes threw my ears. Damn no pushing away my fears anymore. These fears are staring me right in the face and there letting me know that my intracranial pressure is high again.I can't win for losing. I guess I should be thankful for the four months I had of peace but the disfunction this disease has caused in my life is just too much. I keep my headache to myself for a couple days to make sure its not going away and sure enough it didn't end. I told my mom and Shane a couple days later. My mom was devastated even though she did her best to hide it. Shane did what he always does and was just there which for some reason always made me feel better. We all tried not to worry, at least until we went to the doctor but we all knew something was wrong.

Chapter Seven

"In diversity there is beauty and there is strength"-Maya Angelou

Something was very wrong. From September until December I underwent countless spinal taps, blood work, MRI'S and CT Scans. NOTHING, the doctors didn't have any answers at all as to why I was having issues yet again. I was miserable. I was back to spending most of my days in bed in pain. My head pounded so hard that if my mouth was closed I could hear my teeth clanking against each other. My ears swooshed so loudly it's all I ever heard. The easiest of task were harder because my head felt like it was trying to escape through my eyeballs. As hard as it was I pushed through, everyday. No matter how long it took the out of state doctors to accept my case or my Neurosurgeon here to find out why I was miserable, I would keep fighting.

I remember the exact moment I accepted the fact that I might be this way forever. I was out to eat with Shane. As we were eating it just seemed like everything slowed down. I was sitting in my wheelchair thinking about how much it had taken for me to be able to go out that night. Shane had to help me shower, help me get dressed, help me to the car on my walker and I sat uncomfortable dreading the outing on the inside. I couldn't do anything else for the entire day to save enough energy for my date and still sitting in this fun restaurant that I once thoroughly enjoyed coming to, I was miserable. But I sat there watching everyone move through their dining experience with smiles and enjoying family. I can barely hear Shane over my head pounding, ears swooshing and pain all over my body. In that moment I made the decision that I would continue to try and get as healthy as I possibly could. Even if after and through this battle I wasn't better, I would keep going. I may have to live the rest of my life in some form of pain but I would try not to focus on the pain but the pleasures life had offered me inspite of the pain. I faced my man and let him know that I loved him, I couldn't stop looking at him, thinking about how blessed I was, mad at myself for not focusing on him in the first place, on our love on how grateful I was to have someone by my side no matter this illness, no matter the pain. Through the months of non stop pain, I focused on my loved ones and the moments I could enjoy. I've had a continuous headache now for a year.

The head pain and swooshing in my ear preserved. In June I added another type of pain to my repertoire. I got out of my bed to use the bathroom when a sharp stabbing,stinging pain brought me to my knees. When I say brought me to my knees I meant literally brought me to my knees. I fell to the ground, hunched over grabbing my side where my shunt is. Ugh the pain was intense but it didn't last long. I hurried to the bathroom and back to lay down in the bed. The pain didn't bother me the rest of the day so I thought nothing else of it. Coming in from outside the next day with my puppy…. BOOM, the pain comes again. It seemed worse than yesterday. The next day with my grandma visiting the house it happens again when I am trying to get out of bed. Im humiliated because Im instantly in tears everytime the pain hits. It sucks that this time people were watching. After about a minute the pain passes and I get back in the bed. My mom tells me that if the pain persist she is taking me to the hospital.

And she did 2 days later. We waited 3 hours in the ER at until I couldn't take it anymore. I was so uncomfortable and the longer I was up the more that pain punched me in the gut. I asked if we could leave and go to a different hospital. My amazing support team agreed and we went to another local Hospital. The hospital seen us quickly and ran all the normal test that I have all the time. The ER doctor thought I might have pancreatitis but I knew in my mind that something was wrong with my shunt. No medicine was helping with the pain so after the test did not reveal anything we went home. I made an appointment with my neurosurgeon and dealt with the pain until then. Of course as always my doctor runs the same test and doesn't find anything. He tries changing my shunt and it takes over 2 hours to change the setting. Normally it only takes 10 minutes at the most, this was confirmation for me that something was wrong with the shunt. I felt crazy to be in the place where I am begging for someone to cut me open and fix whatever was ailing me but the pain was that bad.

Reluctantly my doctor agreed to do surgery. He said it is possible that the tubing in my stomache is causing adhesions. That is when scar tissue attaches itself to the tubing. He said he could go in and break up the adhesions and ensure everything was okay.That made sense to me, I mean my incision on my stomach had been reopened in 5 different surgeries. A few days later I had my seventh surgery. I wasn't nervous or scared or anything like that I was just ready. Ready for this pain to stop. The surgery was short it only took about an hour. When I woke up and heard what Dr.McConnel had found I was validated because my thoughts were correct. Something had been wrong with my shunt. When Dr.McConnel opened me up he found that in one of the two places where my shunt was supposed to be attached, it was unattached and it had started wrapping around itself. That was the pain I was feeling, that little thing that probably wouldn't affect most people was bringing me to my knees. But it was over thank God.

Chapter Eight

"Being able to walk pain-free is a blessing. Being able to walk without showing the pain is a skill"-Kyle McPherson

It's now August of 2017 just a couple months after surgery number 7 when we get a letter in the mail saying Dr.Lucca at Johns Hopkins Hospital in Baltimore Maryland has agreed to take me on as a patient. They set up all these appointments for the end of August. As happy as we were about the news it was also met with sadness because I had just had surgery I couldn't physically make this trip right now. And we can't afford it at the moment.As my headaches continue to get worse and keep me from sleeping, my mom works her mommy magic like she always does. After days of her talking to the hospital,they agreed to move back our appointments for a couple months. Once they moved my appointments we started making travel plans for november. That would be when my whole world could change. It was going to be a long hard 7 hour trip to Baltimore but it was going to be worth it.

On November 13th,2017 me with my mom and our close family friend Ms.Rhonda in tow, we started our road trip to Baltimore. We rented a truck, got us some snacks and headed out. There was beautiful weather and we were jamming to our music throughout the entire trip. We turned a 7 hour trip into 9 and Frequently we had to stop. I kept needing to stretch and use the bathroom, I hated that it made the trip longer but we did what we needed too. I was so anxious to meet this doctor, even if he couldn't help entirely, anything he could do would be better than where I was now. Even though I was anxious I was sad too. I had this thought in the back of my mind that Dr.Lucca may not be able to help me. That would mean we spent all this money and people took off work for nothing. More importantly that would mean no change for me.And that was a reality I wasn't ready to face.

He did help though, immensely. Dr.Lucca performed all the normal test they do at home, CT Scans, MRI,x rays. He also performed nuclear test, that weren't available to me at home. In the nuclear test they injected nuclear dye into my shunts. Then a few hours later they perform imaging that shows the flow of the dye through my shunt tubes. From that testing the doctor was able to tell us that one of my shunts was partially obstructed. He also was able to see that I had developed a Chiari Malformation.Chiari Malformation is when brain tissue extends into your spinal canal. Normally this happens because of a small opening in your skull but this can occur in people with different conditions if the spinal pressure in the brain becomes to low. That is what happened with me. My shunts not working properly was draining too much fluid and caused brain tissue to start extending into my spinal canal. The chiari was causing all the pain in my neck and shoulders,the dizziness and adding to the headache, the blockage was probably causing the rest of my symptoms and adding to my headache. I was relieved, so relieved I cried sitting right there in the doctor's office. I had been fighting for over a year to get my doctor to just pay attention to me and my symptoms, just to do testing and tell me if I was crazy or if there was something wrong with me. All I wanted was normalcy and to not have a headache and for a year my doctor told me nothing was wrong with me when in fact there was. Relief, thankfulness and all that pain rolled down my face as I cried. We planned to travel back to Baltimore soon to have a surgical test done that would give him more direction on how to treat me. Now I'm excited. I couldn't wait to call Shane and tell him the good news.

A couple weeks later we got a letter in the mail saying my ICP Bolt Monitoring surgery was scheduled for January 9th. With this test they'd drill a hole in my skull and Insert a bolt that would continuously monitor what my spinal fluid was. While in the hospital they'd monitor me while walking, laying down, sitting up and eating. Oddly enough hearing that I'd have to have yet another brain surgery didn't disappoint me I was happy and ready. I had brought this test to my doctor's here in Columbus and he refused to do it so I couldn't wait.

This time when we went to Johns Hopkins we would fly. Flying is quicker and would be easier on me physically when we have to return home after my procedure. Shane, my mom and I bought our tickets, they took off work and we prepared to leave. All there was to do now was enjoy the holidays and wait.

I always get sentimental and nostalgic before a surgery, because you never know what could happen even with a routine procedure.Let's be honest anytime you go under the knife you could die. Those chances are dramatically increased when someone is poking around your brain.But I couldn't be afraid of dying or of anything I had to enjoy what I could in every moment I could. Watching all the kids in my family at thanksgiving helped me with that. They really made me smile. Eating the amazing meal my mom prepared for Christmas was peaceful to me. Having a drink and some fun on new year's eve was the icing on the cake. Now I was ready to face this surgery head on. Only 8 days left.

January 9th came and we set out for Baltimore. We had to be at the airport at 4:30am. It took us longer to check our luggage, and the wheelchair then it did for the flight. 50 minutes in the air and we were on our way to my new future. Tonight we'd stay in a hotel and at 6am we would head to the hospital. Knowing this procedure was coming had not made me nervous but excited. It may sound odd that I was wishing and excited for a brain surgery but the only alternative was living with the pain I had carried with me for years, and that I could not do!

At 6am Wednesday we drove to the hospital. Immediately I was taking back about how nice everyone was. Registration, and all the nurses were helpful and kind. I was ready for surgery and waiting to meet the doctor, that's when the reality of having my 8th surgery in a few minutes set in. What if this procedure doesn't work like all the other ones? What happens to my support team if I'm not able to be around for them? How crazy will I seem if these results don't match my symptoms? Am I crazy for wanting to come this far to have a surgery, away from my home, my family, my dog? All those questions rolled through my head as my mom prays with us and the surgical nurse. It's showtime now, they give me the happy drugs and roll me away from family. "Can you play some music?" I ask the surgical tech as we enter the sterile and cold operating room. She smiles and ask me what kind of music I like. I tell her anything really but Blake Shelton would be nice.I start smiling when I hear his song "honey bee" playing over the loudspeaker. I sing away as they put me on another table and stabilize my head in the helmet. I guess the nurse could see my anxiety because she simply touched my hand as they prepared for surgery. I hear Dr.Lucca come in and he gave me a comforting touch and I know it's time. Count backwards from ten he said to me 10.... 9, 8.......

I woke up thinking about why I never get past number 8 and I was in so much pain. My head felt like it was being smashed in a compactor. I can feel the nurse inject more medicine in my IV and back to sleep I go. When I wake up the second time I hear teen mom OG on the t.v. and I know my mom is near. I can feel Shane's hand resting on my leg and I know he's there. After every surgery knowing those two are there eases me. My pain is not as bad as I thought and I mumble hey to let them know I am awake. Kisses and hugs from my favorite humans wake me up further. Now I realize I'm hungry.

My family can't believe that I'm up and alert and of course asking for food. I can't believe I have a bolt in my head. The medicine knocks me out so the next couple days I don't remember much. I know all the nurses were exceptional and the room mate I was forced to listen to all night was very loud. Friday morning comes and it's time for my testing. The doctor monitors how my pressure changes at many different angles. When I stand up immediately I can see the concerned look on the doctors face. She makes me lay down and says she has to go get Dr.Lucca. I'm worried because were supposed to be flying home tomorrow. The doctor comes back and tells us that my pressure is extremely low. With two shunts, even with one only partially working my pressure shouldn't be as low as it is. Dr.Lucca thinks there is a leak and wants to do exploratory surgery to find and fix the leak. I look over and see the tears in my moms eyes. She leaves the room, saying she is going to call the airline to change our flight but I know she wants to cry alone. There is nothing but worry on Shane's face, he'll never say it but I know he is as worried as I am. But our worry and fears don't matter because we have to do the surgery and soon. Dr. Lucca plans for me to have surgery number 9 saturday morning.Which was supposed to be the day I could go home. Oh well I have to do this, I can do this.

That night seemed to fly by quickly. I was so nervous I couldn't sleep. All night I watched hulu and talked to the nurses. When morning came around they took me downstairs to wait until I go into the operating room. Oddly enough I was hungry again since I hadn't been able to eat the day before. I meditated while we waited trying to prepare for the pain I was going to experience in a few hours. With a clear mind and calmed heart my mom, Shane and I laughed at old hospital memories while we waited for Dr.Lucca. Like the time my mom was walking up and down the hall at riverside hospital calling a nurse Tammy whose name wasn't tammy. Or the time she left me in a wheelchair in an elevator at a doctor's appointment. Or one of my favorites the video of me singing the proud family theme song when I woke up from a surgery a couple years ago. The pictures Shane draw for me while he's waiting for my surgery to be over. We were laughing so hard we missed when the doctor came in and almost missed our time to pray before they wheeled me off. After we prayed I was off. They played some Blake Shelton for me again and I got on the operating table with my brain bolt still attached.Surgery number nine was about to be underway.

I woke up in more pain than I had ever felt in my life. Oh the muscles in my back felt like they were being shredded by glass shards. It was bad. And the medicine only made a dent in the pain. I had to continue to lay flat because they were still monitoring my pressures with the bolt. All the wires and probes did not aid in my comfort. Either way I moved I felt pain and I couldn't see that changing anytime soon. Laying in the bed my fears took over my thoughts. I circled around how the last time I was in this much pain when I tried to walk I couldn't. I was terrified of how my body would react to the 4th surgery on my spine in just as many years. I layed with those fears and all that pain, wrapped in my own wires not eating and nauseous for the next two days. Monday it was time to test my pressures once again which means I have to get out of bed. As hard as it was with assistance I got up and I walked. Not as well as I had been but I was fine. I asked the doctor if I could get a muscle relaxant to help ease the pain in my muscles. It took them hours to find one that I wasn't allergic to and that would not react with my other medications but once I was able to take one my pain lessened. Based on the testing my pressures were doing better as well. The doctor said my pressures only spiked when I was sleeping and they were nowhere near as low as they were

before. Most importantly though by the grace of God for the first time in two years I did not have a headache.

Whoa! I blow out a sigh of relief while telling my doctor's the excellent news. I see the tears of

happiness in my moms eyes this time. The smile in shanes eye, the relief in the doctor's voice when he

knows he solved one of my problems. Finally. Although we have this good news just to be safe the doctors

keep me one more night to make sure the results of my testing are accurate. Thank goodness they were.

Tuesday morning the team of residents come in and let me know I'm going home. Yayy. I just have one

more battle to get through while I am here. I have to sit awake while they unscrew this bolt in my head and

pull it out, then stitch me up. The doctors don't tell you that tidbit of information when you agree to have this

procedure done. Although I wasn't prepared for this pain, ready or not I was going to face it. It was the only

thing standing in my way of getting on that plane and going home.

I put my big girl panties on, meditated and got pain medication from the nurses. The doctors came in

and covered my face. I could feel the tugging as they pulled the bandages from my adhesive filled hair and

scalp. I started thinking okay maybe this won't be that bad. I quickly found out it would be worse than bad.

The unscrewing started and my body cringes at the pain. It seems as if I can feel the sound of the bolt

unscrewing from my skull. At times I thought I'd pass out. Lucky me, since I have such small ventricles in my

brain they had to put the bolt further in to get readings and now it is kind of stuck. With all the extra pulling

they have to do they give me more medicine. The physicians assistant holds my hand while they pull it out.

I'll never forget that popping sound it made when they pulled it out. Getting the stitch sewed in wasn't as bad

as the rest of this process so we talk while they're finishing up. Last step complete, now I get to go home.

Headache free

We have 6 or so hours before our flight leaves so we go back to the hotel that My mom and shane have been sleeping at during the night. It will be nice to rest before we leave. It feels so good to sleep in a bed without bars and to not have to lay flat. All of us are so happy to be leaving. Were also all exhausted in every way imaginable. Johns Hopkins was amazing and much better than the hospitals I had experienced in Ohio but its not home. After a nap and some food we head to the airport. We had another 50 minute flight to Columbus. With my painkillers and muscle relaxers I knew I could make it even with stitches in my head and down my spine. This week long adventure in Baltimore was almost over and I could practically feel my memory foam mattress. 50 minutes slowly ticks away until it's time to land. The whole time I'm thinking about how none of this, the booking and rebooking of flights, all of my pain, spending the money, and all this stress would have never happened if my doctors at home had just listened to me when I asked about this test years ago.I spent these years not only seeing my neurosurgeon frequently but other doctors he had referred me to as well. Doctor after doctor said my condition wasn't the cause of my headaches. One thought it was a neck issue,another thought I needed botox, another put me on a medicine that gave me mood swings.All I needed was for them to listen. Then I could've spent the last 2 years of my life without the insurmountable amount of pain. What if?

There was no time to think about what ifs though because we had landed in Columbus Ohio. Home. For the next few weeks I did nothing but stay at home. Since I had open wounds especially near my brain I couldn't be around many people so I rested and healed. Even during my healing process I felt better than I had in years. I was sleeping again and still no headache. The pain I had in my shoulders and arms slowly subsided. The tingling in my hands and feet had gone away too. I was back using my cane and I had a strength I couldn't explain. A strength that I had never had. I felt empowered and ready to enjoy this headache free life for as long as I could.

Chapter Nine

"I don't want my pain and struggle to make me a victim.I want my battle to make me someone else's hero."-Unknown

14 days later I go to my primary care physician to get my stitches out. The ones along my spine came out effortlessly but the ones in my head had not dissolved the way they were supposed too so my doctor had to cut them out. That was the easiest and quickest doctors appointment I have had since 2014. Now that my wounds are closed up I start going out and about more. The freedom of no headache I had taken for granted. I had forgotten what it felt like to do things without head pain. I wasn't pain free completely and probably will never be but this pain is tolerable.Even more so without my head trying to escape through my eyes and ears everyday all day long.

The next few weeks were spent getting acclimated to my new normal. I started doing my therapy exercises again. I caught up on all the sleep I had missed. I was walking almost exclusively on my cane. I was having fun again. People commented on how different I looked, how my smile was different. I was actually getting excited and less anxious about this new normal I was in. I'd feel totally secure that everything was okay once we went and seen Dr.Lucca at Johns Hopkins again. My follow up appointment was in a couple weeks and I was prepared for whatever would come at this appointment. This time it would be just me and my mom, we would fly out and back home all in the same day. Hopefully unlike our last visit we wouldn't have to stay longer than intended.

Thank goodness we didn't have to stay. Our appointment went flawlessly. Dr.Lucca said everything looked brilliantly, he just wanted me to get a CT Scan so we can have it as a reference for when things did get bad. That was easy enough for me to handle. Some of my stitches still haven't dissolved so the nurse came in and cut them out for me. As quickly as we got to Baltimore, it was time to leave. We were more than happy.

Chapter Ten

"There is an old saying that what doesn't kill you makes you stronger. I don't

believe that. I think the things that try to kill you make you angry and

sad. Strength comes from the good things. Your family, Your friends, the satisfaction

of hard work. Those are the things that will keep you whole. Those are the things to

hold onto when you're broken." - Jax Teller

The physical things I had gone through and was going through only amplified everything else that was going on because of these illnesses. I had lost my job and my education because of these illnesses, and it was hard for me. I had to humble myself and turn to the government for help. I had decided to apply for social security disability.

That process was horrendous. My application was denied 4 times in 2 years. While denying me, social security made me go see countless doctor's. Twice they made me see a psychiatrist. They thought I was crazy. Once they said my application was denied for me not being blind enough although I was legally blind. Then they denied me because epilepsy was not enough of a disability to them. I never figured out why they denied me the 3rd or 4th time but they didn't even have Pseudotumor Cerebri listed as my diagnosis on my application. It made me immensely grateful for the financial help I got from my mom and my boyfriend. Why is it so hard for people who need the help to get the help. I've worked and paid into social security since I was 15 years old, now that I need to draw from it, I'm being told no. It was beyond frustrating. At times I just wanted to give up. I was sick and tired of being sick tired and broke with no way of supporting myself. But just when I thought I would give up on applying, a friend told me about an attorney who had helped him get approved for disability. I contacted her that evening and the next week she came to my house and explained the long tedious process of applying for assistance. She explained I could ask for a hearing after so many denials so that a judge could determine if I needed disability. Mrs.Jacobson told us it might be a long process but she has had success in similar circumstances. We hired her that day, and I am so glad we did because a little over a year later I was ordered by a judge full disability benefits and back pay from the very first time I was denied in 2014. I was so excited and relieved. Finally. The feeling of being able to take care of myself again was unmatched.

It wasn't just the financial strain either mentally I was struggling as well. I was struggling with the fact that my memory was slipping away. I was stricken with the pain of feeling nothing but pain. I was numb to everything around me. I was tired of all the medications and side effects. I felt trapped in a body that wasn't the body I remembered. I had to deal with the grief of losing myself while still having to smile and go on with life. When you grieve the death of a loved one other people understand, its okay to stay in bed a couple days and cry, no one understands grief of yourself, your own life when your technically still living it. Not only that I had to deal with everything that came with the pseudotumor, while dealing with the possibility of having a seizure at any moment.. Which happened more than a few times during this journey of mine.What was I supposed to do other than grin and bear it. Tell others I was okay when I wasn't. Just having to lie all the time to everyone simply because they couldn't take knowing how much pain you were really in. I hated myself sometimes for wishing for the pain just so that I could know I was alive.I struggled with the fear that I may die at anytime from any one of the conditions I had. Mentally I was struggling no matter how well I dealt with it, how much I prayed or meditated, I had bad days and I was exhausted in every sense of the word. Eventually and sadly I got used to the mental struggle, writing, talking, and helping others with Pseudotumor, took away a lot of the mental stress that came with my chronic illnesses. When I started writing, I came across a story of an old woman wishing people enough. She explained to whomever she is telling this story, that when her family says I wish you enough they're wishing that person enough good things in life to sustain them. Enough sun to keep them bright,enough rain to appreciate the sun, enough happiness to keep their spirit alive,enough pain to appreciate the joys,enough gain to satisfy your wanting, enough loss to appreciate what you posses and enough hellos to appreciate the goodbyes.Writing and helping others gave me enough to be okay.

Chapter eleven

"When your faith is tested, Endurance can grow." James 1:3 nkjv

Although the last four years of my life have been a battlefield, I wouldn't trade them for the world. If Pseudotumor has taught me anything it's that no matter the obstacle or opponent you can get through it,the peace and understanding that I have gained knowing that and everything else I've learned is unmatched to anything I would have experienced otherwise. I use to have these sad realization moments where I'd realize a sad fact about my new chronically ill life and cry.For example when i fell over the vacuum in my living room one night. Sad realization was that night blindness is a real thing when your losing your vision because of Pseudotumor Cerebri. I cried laying over the vacuum, that has been in the same spot in the same living room I had lived in all of my life. How could I fall? Am I never going to be able to see in the dark again? Well no! I still can't see in the dark but the moment or moments like that don't make me sad anymore. Listening to one of my favorite musicians Lyfe Jennings the next day, I remembered that no matter what the sad realization was in my life it could always be worse. No I can't stand without holding onto something or someone but at least I can stand, yes I am exhausted from everyday activities but at least I woke up and can do those activities. I didn't think that way before my illness. Before everything to me had to be perfect.If it wasn't perfect just like I planned it then it didn't matter That is never the case with a chronic illness. And I learned that the hard way.

These illnesses also taught me to be brutally honest with myself and self evaluate my feelings. No matter what the doctor said, or how I felt physically I tried to be honest with myself about how I felt emotionally. I knew it would be the only way I would make it through. When I was still trying to drive and go to work knowing I was half blind and hurting I had to be honest with myself. I acknowledged that working wasn't the best option and I needed to lay my ass back down. The honesty with myself helped me do what I needed to do when i needed it. Self awareness allowed me to put my health first no matter how much being in denial was easier.

Changing how I looked at life helped me manage the battle as well. Before my illness I worked two jobs, I danced competitively, i skated twice a week. I didn't have much time for a social life but I didn't care because my goals were all that mattered. Being that way comes with sacrifices though and I missed a lot. I missed times with my niece, and family event's, I missed the enjoyment of having fun and relaxation.Enjoying myself and quiet. I missed finding what else fulfilled me or could make me happy. Now I cant skate or even dance like I used too, but I learned that cooking is something I love. I even taught myself how to crochet. I'm not very good at crocheting but I enjoy it immensely. Shane taught me how to fish and that's something we enjoy together now. Gardening made me look at nature in a whole different light but planting and watching your own food grow is rewarding in a way I could have ever imagined. Also I'm teaching myself a new language and to play the guitar. Which I've always wanted to do but never had the time. To begin to enjoy the new things I now love I had to stop looking at my ill life as a burden but a blessing in disguise. A blessing that hurt but allowed me to learn more about myself and to become a more rounded person, a better person. The best part of changing my outlook is even though it hurt like hell it changed my life for the better! I will be always be grateful for that.

Chapter twelve

"If I cannot do great things. I can do small things in a great way"- Dr. Martin Luther King Jr.

I took for granted how much energy it takes to be sick. It seems like I am always exhausted. There were days and days where I never even left my house, I could only make it out of my bed to pee. When that is what your life is reduced to, you take advantage of the times you feel better. I was inpatient before my illness but now it seems to be worse.If I feel well enough to do it or have it, I take it. Why wait for anything. Being chronically ill you never know what tomorrow could be like. In 10 mins I could have had a seizure and be on my way to the hospital, I could be having surgery tomorrow or worse, dead. So if there is something i want I do it. Right then. I guess the old saying is true, why wait to do tomorrow what you can do today. Remembering that helped me take advantage of every moment during this battle, good or bad. Do what you can while you can, get what you want, when you want it.

People who know my story always tell me how strong I am. There were times in the thick of my battle where I forgot how strong I was. There were times when I was to weak to even fight for myself. My doctors had given up and so did I. But my mom always fought for me and with me. In ways she doesn't know. Things as simple as playing her favorite gospel CD by Kirk Franklin "Losing My Religion". When I would ride with her in the car listening to those songs they helped me. The most important was the song where Kirk Franklin says "while your waiting on the blessing you want, don't forget the blessing you are." And something clicked for me. My life is a blessing, the simple fact that I'm alive is a testimony. I have survived brain surgeries, it doesn't matter that I am not what I was just that I am here to keep trying to get there. I have to remember that fact when I'm too weak to stand up to those doctors. Yes I'm a blessing and I have to keep fighting to get the blessing that's coming to me. When I wake up from surgeries, when my pain is at its worse I tell myself that, I repeat in my head "I am a blessing, I'm here and I am a blessing" Even in the thick of the battle don't forget the blessing you are.

Remembering my blessings wasn't the only thing that helped me through in the pain peppered times, fighting for myself did too. No matter what the doctors told me I did my own research. I kept looking for help from other doctors, looking for cures and treatments anywhere I could find them. I talked to anyone who would listen. I kept fighting. I am still fighting. It took two years of having unimaginable head pain that I didn't need to endure but I did until I got help and now I can say that I am better. The validation of fighting for what you need and getting it, is amazing. What if I had given up entirely, I would have never gotten the help I needed. I would still have the head pain. I would still be miserable.I wouldn't be better. Don't be miserable when all you have to do is fight. Fight for you! Even if nothing comes from it, it is worth it.

When I think about how bad things got for me I always think about how much worse it would've been if I would have had to go through this by myself. When I got sick it showed me who my real friends are and even showed which family members I could truly depend on. There are people with my conditions and worse who go through it all alone. My man and my mom never even missed a doctor appointment with me.They were always there. Always having them around made me realize how very special family and love can be. Now I try to tell my loved ones how special they are to me everyday. I want them to hear me tell them I love them while I can still say it. I need them to know now that they are the biggest blessing in the world to me. Your love ones should know that they are appreciated for all that they do whether you are sick or not. I am thankful that my illness as terrible as it is taught me to love in a deeper way to love the people that mean the most to me with all my might.

The biggest part of dealing with this chronic illness thing is learning to stay calm. As strong as I think I am, as calm as I am , I always get nervous right before its time for surgery. Prayer and meditation aided in keeping me calm. I pray all the time and that helps but it's something about meditation that clears my mind and calms my heart. I meditate before going to the hospital and it puts me at peace when I need it. Sometimes clearing your mind helps you focus without you really focusing, it takes your mind off of what is in front of you so you can get through what is in front of you ,without worrying about it. Pray, meditate and go forth because when you get down to it we honestly don't have any other choice but to go on!

Whenever I'm in the hospital I always take pictures, not because I'm vain but because I want to remember every moment I can so I'll never forget. My last surgery when I posted my ugly pictures with the bolt in my head and my hair missing someone from my Pseudotumor Support Group messaged me and said how much seeing my pictures had meant to her. She hadnt had surgery yet and was newly diagnosed but seeing me smile in the hospital gave her hope. That warmed my heart, even when I'm in pain I try to smile, in the hospital I smile because you don't know who that smile is affecting, who might see the brightness in you and it brightens something in their life. Life may suck but smile anyway. Hospital memories suck most times but their mine.Seeing myself smile makes any problem a little easier to deal with it. You'd be dealing with the same problem if you didn't smile so you might as well smile. Even if you don't smile for yourself do it for someone else! Smile anyway!

My illnesses will not ever go away. Although I am better, Im still in pain everyday. I still fall over if I stand longer than a few minutes without holding something, I still can't shower alone and my shunts hurt sometimes.I still never hear silence, My ears rings and swoosh all the time. My neck still aches at times and I still feel one of the pieces of my broken plastic shunt tearing through my back muscles. And most annoyingly I am always tired but most importantly I'm better. Although I have issues I enjoy things in my life and the people in it. Because of my conditions I have a new found love for myself and I can share with others the things I've learned during this crazy battle.Because of this battle, I have new goals, new dreams and as a patient advocate I get to help people everyday.Before my illness I worked in healthcare and I loved helping and caring for people. My dream was to get my masters in Gerontology and healthcare administration.I wanted to use that degree to make healthcare better for the elderly. Although I can not help people in the same way anymore, I will still make a difference to people who need it. My new goal will help people who endure like me everyday. I want to start a nonprofit foundation called Enduring Minds. I've been planning it for a couple years now, this book and my blog were steps to making that dream a reality. Enduring Minds the foundation will provide patient advocacy, educational support,counseling, and financial help for those who endure life with a rare chronic illness that affects the mind. Conditions like mine and hopefully one day countless others. I want to most importantly raise awareness and always be working towards a cure but until that is possible, I want to help us keep enduring everyday. It may not be the life or career I planned but its mine and it will make a difference and I am so excited about it. They say if you want to make God laugh tell him what you got planned. I guess he is up in heaven with my grandfather laughing at my past plans as my purpose in this life is now being fulfilled. Until a cure comes along or I am no longer able I will keep fighting, keep helping where I can and enjoying all the bad and good that comes my way. Everyone has a cross to bare, this is just mine. God thought I was Bad Ass enough to handle this battle and finally I do too!!

THE END

AFTERWORD:

Dear Amorcito,

Thank you for standing with me and loving me through it all. I can not put into words how much I love and appreciate you. You are my best friend, the love of my life and my superman. I will spend every day that I draw breath working to make you the happiest man alive. To the only person who can make my heart beat faster and slower at the same time, I am so in love with you. None of this would be possible without your support.

I want to thank every single person who has supported my writing. From reading my blog and sharing my work on The Mighty to now reading my first published novel. It means so very much to me and my family. I want everyone to know that supporting me by reading this book will be supporting a lot of others as well. All of the proceeds from this book will be used to start my non-profit foundation Enduring Minds. This foundation will raise awareness for rare and chronic brain conditions such as Intracranial Hypertension and Epilepsy. Also it will give scholarships to students pursuing their education while enduring and offer advice, patient advocacy and assistance to those who endure and need it.

To read more go to www.enduringminds.com

To donate go to https://www.gofundme.com/enduring-minds-the-foundation&rcid=r01-153072180376-7fddcbac69e0476c&pc=ot_co_campmgmt_w

Follow us, Like and Share on all social media @ Enduring Minds

Thank you from the bottom of my heart!!

Doctors names have been changed to protect confidentiality.